Important Phone Numbers

Emergency _____

Clinic _____

Nurse _____

Doctor _____

Other _____

_____

For More Information

This is only one of many free books for people with cancer.
Here are some others you may find useful:

- *Biological Therapy*

- *Radiation Therapy and You: Support for People With Cancer*

- *Eating Hints: Before, During, and After Cancer Treatment*

- *Taking Part in Cancer Treatment Research Studies*

- *Thinking About Complementary & Alternative Medicine:
  A Guide for People With Cancer*

- *Pain Control: A Guide for People With Cancer*

- *When Cancer Returns*

- *Taking Time: Support for People with Cancer*

These books are available from NCI (the National Cancer Institute). NCI is a federal
agency that is part of the National Institutes of Health. Call 1-800-4-CANCER
(1-800-422-6237) or visit www.cancer.gov. (See page 59 for more information.)

For information about your specific type of cancer, see the PDQ database.
You can also find the database at www.cancer.gov.

Product or brand names that appear in this book are for example only. The U.S.
Government does not endorse any specific product or brand. If products or brands
are not mentioned, it does not mean or imply that they are not satisfactory.

About This Book

Chemotherapy and You is written for you—someone who is about to receive or is now receiving **chemotherapy** for cancer. Your family, friends, and others close to you may also want to read this book.

This book is a guide you can refer to throughout your chemotherapy treatment. It includes facts about chemotherapy and its **side effects** and also highlights ways you can care for yourself before, during, and after treatment.

Rather than read this book from beginning to end— look at only those sections you need now. Later, you can always read more.

This book covers:

■ Questions and answers about chemotherapy.
Answers common questions, such as what chemotherapy is and how it affects cancer cells.

■ Side effects and ways to manage them.
Explains side effects and other problems that may result from chemotherapy. This section also has ways that you and your doctor or nurse can manage these side effects.

■ Tips for meeting with your doctor or nurse.
Includes questions for you to think about and discuss with your doctor, nurse, and others involved in your cancer care.

■ Ways to learn more.
Lists ways to get more information about chemotherapy and other topics discussed in this book—in print, online, and by telephone.

■ Words to know.
A dictionary that clearly explains all the words that are in bold in this book.

Talk with your doctor or nurse about what you can expect during chemotherapy. He or she may suggest that you read certain sections of this book or try some of the ways to manage side effects.

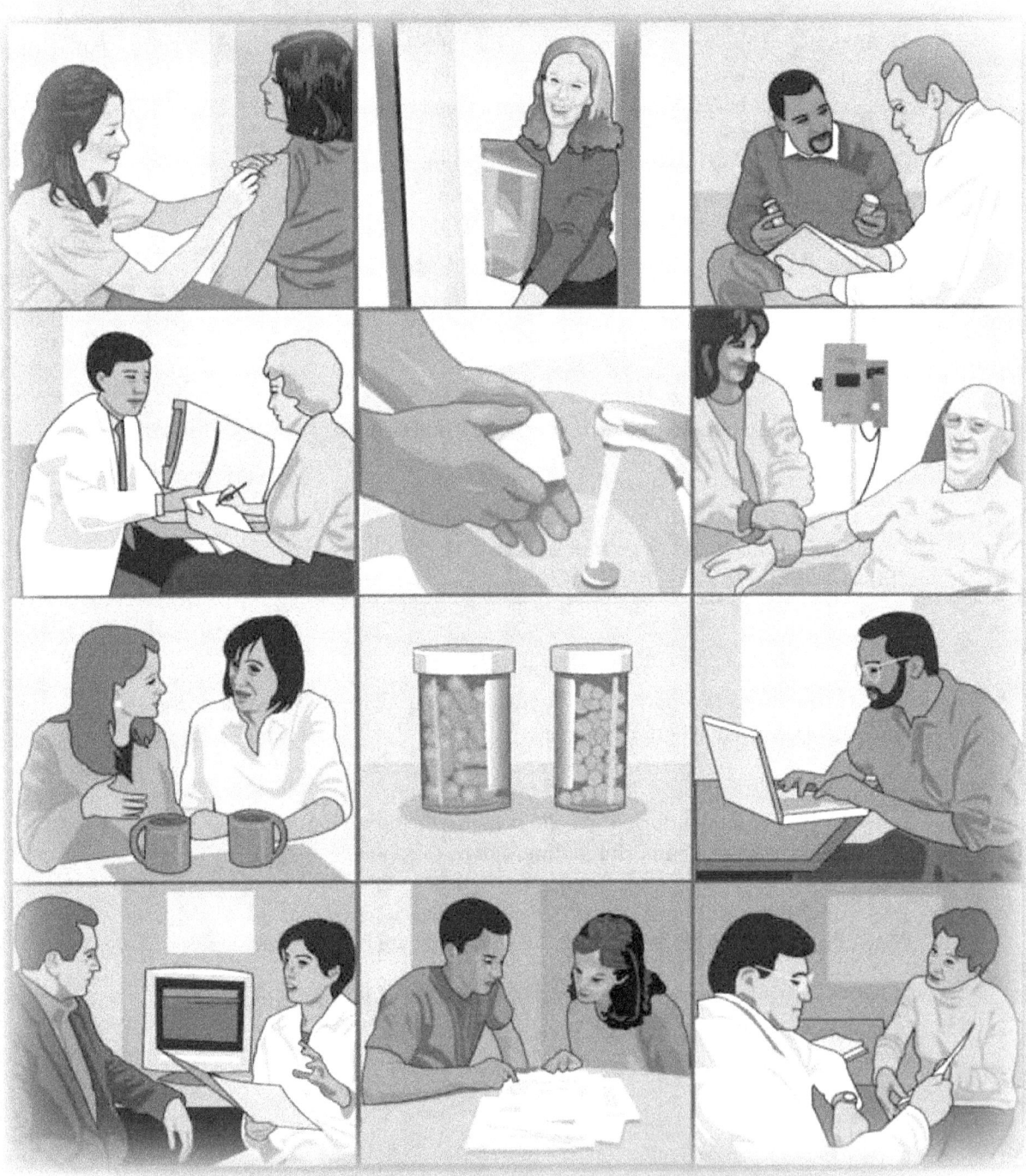

Table of Contents

Rather than read this book from beginning to end— <u>look at only those sections you need now.</u> Later, you can always read more.

What is chemotherapy?	Chemotherapy (also called chemo) is a type of cancer treatment that uses drugs to destroy cancer cells.
How does chemotherapy work?	Chemotherapy works by stopping or slowing the growth of cancer cells, which grow and divide quickly. But it can also harm **healthy cells** that divide quickly, such as those that line your mouth and intestines or cause your hair to grow. Damage to healthy cells may cause side effects. Often, side effects get better or go away after chemotherapy is over.
What does chemotherapy do?	Depending on your type of cancer and how advanced it is, chemotherapy can:

- Cure cancer—when chemotherapy destroys cancer cells to the point that your doctor can no longer detect them in your body and they will not grow back.

- Control cancer—when chemotherapy keeps cancer from spreading, slows its growth, or destroys cancer cells that have spread to other parts of your body.

- Ease cancer symptoms (also called **palliative care**)—when chemotherapy shrinks tumors that are causing pain or pressure.

How is chemotherapy used?	Sometimes, chemotherapy is used as the only cancer treatment. But more often, you will get chemotherapy along with surgery, **radiation therapy**, or **biological therapy**. Chemotherapy can:

- Make a tumor smaller before surgery or radiation therapy. This is called **neo-adjuvant chemotherapy**.

- Destroy cancer cells that may remain after surgery or radiation therapy. This is called **adjuvant chemotherapy**.

- Help radiation therapy and biological therapy work better.

- Destroy cancer cells that have come back (**recurrent** cancer) or spread to other parts of your body (**metastatic** cancer).

How does my doctor decide which chemotherapy drugs to use?	This choice depends on: ▪ The type of cancer you have. Some types of chemotherapy drugs are used for many types of cancer. Other drugs are used for just one or two types of cancer. ▪ Whether you have had chemotherapy before. ▪ Whether you have other health problems, such as diabetes or heart disease.
Where do I go for chemotherapy?	You may receive chemotherapy during a hospital stay, at home, or in a doctor's office, clinic, or **outpatient** unit in a hospital (which means you do not have to stay overnight). No matter where you go for chemotherapy, your doctor and nurse will watch for side effects and make any needed drug changes.
How often will I receive chemotherapy?	Treatment schedules for chemotherapy vary widely. How often and how long you get chemotherapy depends on: ▪ Your type of cancer and how advanced it is ▪ The goals of treatment (whether chemotherapy is used to cure your cancer, control its growth, or ease the symptoms) ▪ The type of chemotherapy ▪ How your body reacts to chemotherapy You may receive chemotherapy in cycles. A cycle is a period of chemotherapy treatment followed by a period of rest. For instance, you might receive 1 week of chemotherapy followed by 3 weeks of rest. These 4 weeks make up one cycle. The rest period gives your body a chance to build new healthy cells.
Can I miss a dose of chemotherapy?	It is not good to skip a chemotherapy treatment. But sometimes your doctor or nurse may change your chemotherapy schedule. This can be due to side effects you are having. If this happens, your doctor or nurse will explain what to do and when to start treatment again.

How is chemotherapy given?

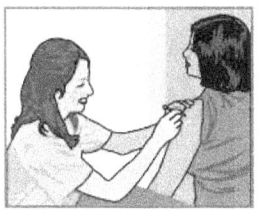

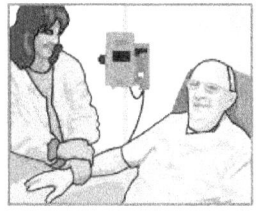

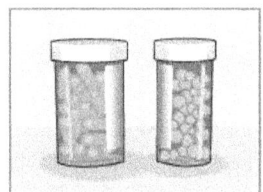

Chemotherapy may be given in many ways.

- **Injection**. The chemotherapy is given by a shot in a muscle in your arm, thigh, or hip, or right under the skin in the fatty part of your arm, leg, or belly.

- **Intra-arterial (IA)**. The chemotherapy goes directly into the artery that is feeding the cancer.

- **Intraperitoneal (IP)**. The chemotherapy goes directly into the **peritoneal cavity** (the area that contains organs such as your intestines, stomach, liver, and ovaries).

- **Intravenous (IV)**. The chemotherapy goes directly into a vein.

- Topical. The chemotherapy comes in a cream that you rub onto your skin.

- Oral. The chemotherapy comes in pills, capsules, or liquids that you swallow.

Things to know about getting chemotherapy through an IV

Chemotherapy is often given through a thin needle that is placed in a vein on your hand or lower arm. Your nurse will put the needle in at the start of each treatment and remove it when treatment is over. Let your doctor or nurse know right away if you feel pain or burning while you are getting IV chemotherapy.

IV chemotherapy is often given through **catheters** or **ports**, sometimes with the help of a **pump**.

■ Catheters. A catheter is a soft, thin tube. A surgeon places one end of the catheter in a large vein, often in your chest area. The other end of the catheter stays outside your body. Most catheters stay in place until all your chemotherapy treatments are done. Catheters can also be used for drugs other than chemotherapy and to draw blood. Be sure to watch for signs of infection around your catheter. For more information on infection, see page 30.

■ Ports. A port is a small, round disc made of plastic or metal that is placed under your skin. A catheter connects the port to a large vein, most often in your chest.

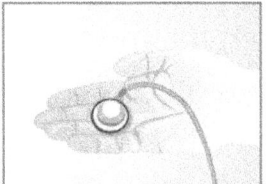
Your nurse can insert a needle into your port to give you chemotherapy or draw blood. This needle can be left in place for chemotherapy treatments that are given for more than 1 day. Be sure to watch for signs of infection around your port. For more information on infection, see page 30.

■ Pumps. Pumps are often attached to catheters or ports. They control how much and how fast chemotherapy goes into a catheter or port. Pumps can be internal or

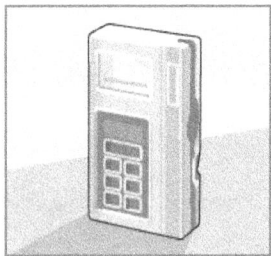
external. External pumps remain outside your body. Most people can carry these pumps with them. Internal pumps are placed under your skin during surgery.

How will I feel during chemotherapy?

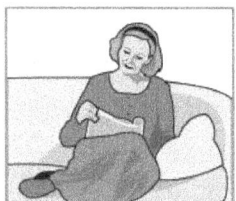

Chemotherapy affects people in different ways. How you feel depends on how healthy you are before treatment, your type of cancer, how advanced it is, the kind of chemotherapy you are getting, and the dose. Doctors and nurses cannot know for certain how you will feel during chemotherapy.

Some people do not feel well right after chemotherapy. The most common side effect is **fatigue**, feeling exhausted and worn out. You can prepare for fatigue by:

- Asking someone to drive you to and from chemotherapy

- Planning time to rest on the day of and day after chemotherapy

- Getting help with meals and childcare the day of and at least 1 day after chemotherapy

There are many ways you can help manage chemotherapy side effects. For more information, see the Side Effects At-A-Glance section starting on page 15.

Can I work during chemotherapy?

Many people can work during chemotherapy, as long as they match their schedule to how they feel. Whether or not you can work may depend on what kind of work you do. If your job allows, you may want to see if you can work part-time or work from home on days you do not feel well.

Many employers are required by law to change your work schedule to meet your needs during cancer treatment. Talk with your employer about ways to adjust your work during chemotherapy. You can learn more about these laws by talking with a social worker.

Can I take over-the-counter and prescription drugs while I get chemotherapy?

This depends on the type of chemotherapy you get and the other types of drugs you plan to take. Take only drugs that are approved by your doctor or nurse. Tell your doctor or nurse about all the over-the-counter and prescription drugs you take, including laxatives, allergy medicines, cold medicines, pain relievers, aspirin, and ibuprofen.

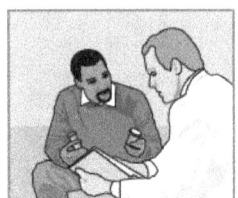

One way to let your doctor or nurse know about these drugs is by bringing in all your pill bottles. Your doctor or nurse needs to know:

- The name of each drug
- The reason you take it
- How much you take
- How often you take it

Talk to your doctor or nurse before you take any over-the-counter or prescription drugs, vitamins, minerals, dietary supplements, or herbs.

Can I take vitamins, minerals, dietary supplements, or herbs while I get chemotherapy?

Some of these products can change how chemotherapy works. For this reason, it is important to tell your doctor or nurse about all the vitamins, minerals, dietary supplements, and herbs that you take before you start chemotherapy. During chemotherapy, talk with your doctor before you take any of these products.

How will I know if my chemotherapy is working?

Your doctor will give you physical exams and medical tests (such as blood tests and x-rays). He or she will also ask you how you feel.

You cannot tell if chemotherapy is working based on its side effects. Some people think that severe side effects mean that chemotherapy is working well, or that no side effects mean that chemotherapy is not working. The truth is that side effects have nothing to do with how well chemotherapy is fighting your cancer.

| How much does chemotherapy cost? | It is hard to say how much chemotherapy will cost. It depends on: |

It is hard to say how much chemotherapy will cost. It depends on:

- The types and doses of chemotherapy used

- How long and how often chemotherapy is given

- Whether you get chemotherapy at home, in a clinic or office, or during a hospital stay

- The part of the country where you live

Does my health insurance pay for chemotherapy?

Talk with your health insurance company about what costs it will pay for. Questions to ask include:

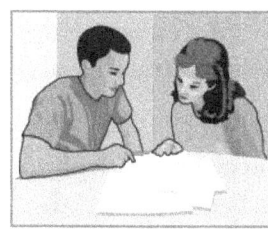

- What will my insurance pay for?

- Do I need to call my insurance company before each treatment for it to be covered? Or, does my doctor's office need to call?

- What do I have to pay for?

- Can I see any doctor I want or do I need to choose from a list of preferred providers?

- Do I need a written referral to see a specialist?

- Is there a co-pay (money I have to pay) each time I have an appointment?

- Is there a deductible (certain amount I need to pay) before my insurance pays?

- Where should I get my prescription drugs?

- Does my insurance pay for all my tests and treatments, whether I am an inpatient or outpatient?

How can I best work with my insurance plan?	▪ Read your insurance policy before treatment starts to find out what your plan will and will not pay for.
	▪ Keep records of all your treatment costs and insurance claims.
	▪ Send your insurance company all the paperwork it asks for. This may include receipts from doctors' visits, prescriptions, and lab work. Be sure to also keep copies for your own records.
	▪ As needed, ask for help with the insurance paperwork. You can ask a friend, family member, social worker, or local group such as a senior center.
	▪ If your insurance does not pay for something you think it should, find out why the plan refused to pay. Then talk with your doctor or nurse about what to do next. He or she may suggest ways to appeal the decision or other actions to take.

| What are clinical trials and are they an option for me? | **Cancer clinical trials** (also called cancer treatment studies or research studies) test new treatments for people with cancer. These can be studies of new types of chemotherapy, other types of treatment, or new ways to combine treatments. The goal of all these clinical trials is to find better ways to help people with cancer. |

Your doctor or nurse may suggest you take part in a clinical trial. You can also suggest the idea. Before you agree to be in a clinical trial, learn about:

▪ Benefits. All clinical trials offer quality cancer care. Ask how this clinical trial could help you or others. For instance, you may be one of the first people to get a new treatment or drug.

▪ Risks. New treatments are not always better or even as good as **standard treatments**. And even if this new treatment is good, it may not work well for you.

▪ Payment. Your insurance company may or may not pay for treatment that is part of a clinical trial. Before you agree to be in a trial, check with your insurance company to make sure it will pay for this treatment.

Contact the NCI's Cancer Information Service if you are interested in learning more about clinical trials. See Ways To Learn More on page 59 for ways to contact them.

■ **Make a list of your questions before each appointment.**
Some people keep a "running list" and write down new
questions as they think of them. Make sure to have space on
this list to write down the answers from your doctor or nurse.

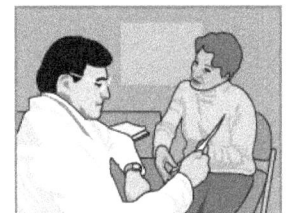

■ **Bring a family member or trusted friend to your medical
visits.** This person can help you understand what the doctor
or nurse says and talk with you about it after the visit is over.

■ **Ask all your questions.** There is no such thing as a stupid question. If you do not
understand an answer, keep asking until you do.

■ **Take notes.** You can write them down or use a tape recorder. Later, you can review your
notes and remember what was said.

■ **Ask for printed information about your type of cancer and chemotherapy.**

■ **Let your doctor or nurse know how much information you want to know, when
you want to learn it, and when you have learned enough.** Some people want to
learn everything they can about cancer and its treatment. Others only want a little
information. The choice is yours.

■ **Find out how to contact your doctor or nurse in an emergency.** This includes who
to call and where to go. Write important phone numbers in the spaces provided on the
inside front cover of this book.

Questions To Ask

**About
My Cancer**

■ What kind of cancer do I have?_____

_____

■ What is the stage of my cancer? _____

_____

**About
Chemotherapy**

■ Why do I need chemotherapy? _____

_____

■ What is the goal of this chemotherapy?_____

_____

■ What are the benefits of chemotherapy? _____

_____

■ What are the risks of chemotherapy? _____

_____

▪ Are there other ways to treat my type of cancer? _____
_____

▪ What is the standard care for my type of cancer? _____
_____

▪ Are there any clinical trials for my type of cancer? _____
_____

About My Treatment

▪ How many cycles of chemotherapy will I get? How long is each treatment? How long between treatments? _____
_____

▪ What types of chemotherapy will I get? _____
_____

▪ How will these drugs be given? _____
_____

▪ Where do I go for this treatment? _____
_____

▪ How long does each treatment last? _____
_____

▪ Should someone drive me to and from treatments? _____
_____

About Side Effects

▪ What side effects can I expect right away? _____
_____

▪ What side effects can I expect later? _____
_____

▪ How serious are these side effects? _____
_____

▪ How long will these side effects last? _____
_____

▪ Will all the side effects go away when treatment is over? _____
_____

▪ What can I do to manage or ease these side effects? _____
_____

▪ What can my doctor or nurse do to manage or ease side effects?
_____

▪ When should I call my doctor or nurse about these side effects?
_____

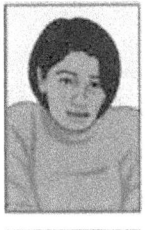
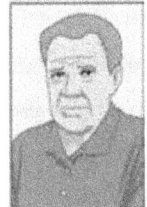
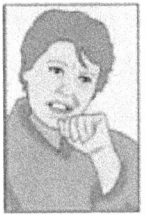
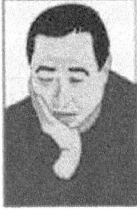

At some point during chemotherapy, you may feel:

- Anxious
- Depressed
- Afraid
- Angry
- Frustrated
- Helpless
- Lonely

It is normal to have a wide range of feelings while going through chemotherapy. After all, living with cancer and getting treatment can be stressful. You may also feel fatigue, which can make it harder to cope with your feelings.

How can I cope with my feelings during chemotherapy?

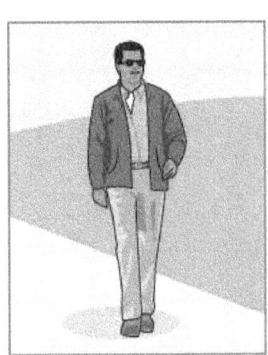

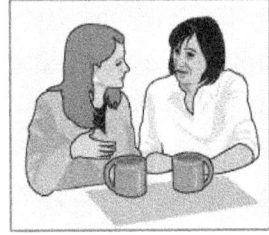

- **Relax.** Find some quiet time and think of yourself in a favorite place. Breathe slowly or listen to soothing music. This may help you feel calmer and less stressed.

- **Exercise.** Many people find that light exercise helps them feel better. There are many ways for you to exercise, such as walking, riding a bike, and doing yoga. Talk with your doctor or nurse about ways you can exercise.

- **Talk with others.** Talk about your feelings with someone you trust. Choose someone who can focus on you, such as a close friend, family member, chaplain, nurse, or social worker. You may also find it helpful to talk with someone else who is getting chemotherapy.

- **Join a support group.** Cancer support groups provide support for people with cancer. These groups allow you to meet others with the same problems. You will have a chance to talk about your feelings and listen to other people talk about theirs. You can find out how others cope with cancer, chemotherapy, and side effects. Your doctor, nurse, or social worker may know about support groups near where you live. Some support groups also meet online (over the Internet), which can be helpful if you cannot travel.

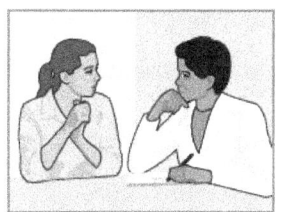

Talk to your doctor or nurse about things that worry or upset you. You may want to ask about seeing a counselor. Your doctor may also suggest that you take medication if you find it very hard to cope with your feelings.

It's normal to have a wide range of feelings during chemotherapy. After all, living with cancer and going through treatment can be stressful.

Ways to learn more

To learn more about coping with your feelings and relationships during cancer treatment, read *Taking Time: Support for People With Cancer*, a book from the National Cancer Institute. You can get a free copy at www.cancer.gov/publications or 1-800-4-CANCER (1-800-422-6237).

Cancer Support Community

Dedicated to providing support, education, and hope to people affected by cancer.

Call:	1-888-793-9355 or 202-659-9709
Visit:	www.cancersupportcommunity.org
E-mail:	help@cancersupportcommunity.org

CancerCare, Inc.

Offers free support, information, financial assistance, and practical help to people with cancer and their loved ones.

Call:	1-800-813-HOPE (1-800-813-4673)
Visit:	www.cancercare.org
E-mail:	info@cancercare.org

Side Effects and Ways To Manage Them

**What are
side effects?**

Side effects are problems caused by cancer treatment. Some
common side effects from chemotherapy are fatigue, **nausea**,
vomiting, decreased **blood cell counts**, hair loss, mouth sores,
and pain.

**What causes
side effects?**

Chemotherapy is designed to kill fast-growing cancer cells.
But it can also affect healthy cells that grow quickly. These include
cells that line your mouth and intestines, cells in your **bone
marrow** that make blood cells, and cells that make your hair
grow. Chemotherapy causes side effects when it harms
these healthy cells.

**Will I get side
effects from
chemotherapy?**

You may have a lot of side effects, some, or none at all. This
depends on the type and amount of chemotherapy you get and
how your body reacts. Before you start chemotherapy, talk with
your doctor or nurse about which side effects to expect.

**How long do
side effects last?**

How long side effects last depends on your health and the
kind of chemotherapy you get. Most side effects go away after
chemotherapy is over. But sometimes it can take months or even
years for them to go away.

Sometimes, chemotherapy causes **long-term side effect**s that
do not go away. These may include damage to your heart, lungs,
nerves, kidneys, or reproductive organs. Some types of chemotherapy may cause a second cancer years later. Ask your doctor or
nurse about your chance of having long-term side effects.

**What can be done
about side effects?**

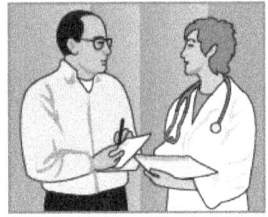

Doctors have many ways to prevent or treat chemotherapy side
effects and help you heal after each treatment session. Talk with
your doctor or nurse about which ones to expect and what to do
about them. Make sure to let your doctor or nurse know about
any changes you notice—they may be signs of a side effect.

The chart on the next page tells you where in this book to look for
more information about specific side effects.

Side Effects At-A-Glance

Below is a list of side effects that chemotherapy may cause.

Not everyone gets every side effect. Which ones you have will depend on the type and dose of your chemotherapy and whether you have other health problems, such as diabetes or heart disease.

You may have a lot of side effects, some, or none at all.

Talk with your doctor or nurse about the side effects on this list. Ask which ones may affect you. Mark the ones you may get and go to the pages listed to learn more.

Names of the chemotherapy that I am getting: _____, _____, _____, _____, _____.

Side effects	Side effects that may affect you	Pages to learn more
Anemia		16
Appetite changes		18
Bleeding		20
Constipation		22
Diarrhea		24
Fatigue		26
Flu-like symptoms		51
Fluid retention		51
Hair loss		28
Infection		30
Infertility		33
Mouth and throat changes		35
Nausea and vomiting		38
Nervous system changes		40
Pain		42
Sexual changes		44
Skin and nail changes		47
Eye changes		51
Urinary, kidney, and bladder changes		50

Anemia

What it is and why it occurs

Red blood cells carry oxygen throughout your body. **Anemia** is when you have too few red blood cells to carry the oxygen your body needs. Your heart works harder when your body does not get enough oxygen. This can make it feel like your heart is pounding or beating very fast. Anemia can also make you feel short of breath, weak, dizzy, faint, or very tired.

Some types of chemotherapy cause anemia because they make it harder for bone marrow to produce new red blood cells.

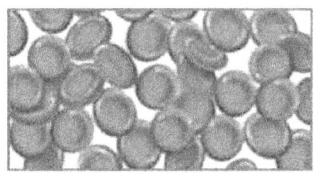

Normal number of red blood cells

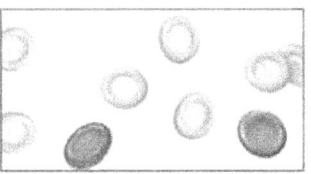

Number of red blood cells when you have anemia

Ways to manage

- **Get plenty of rest.** Try to sleep at least 8 hours each night. You might also want to take 1 to 2 short naps (1 hour or less) during the day.

- **Limit your activities.** This means doing only the activities that are most important to you. For example, you might go to work but not clean the house. Or you might order take-out food instead of cooking dinner.

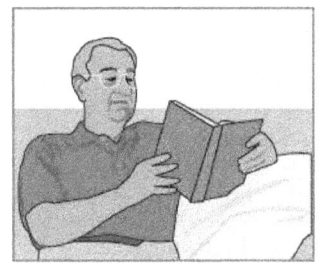

- **Accept help.** When your family or friends offer to help, let them. They can help care for your children, pick up groceries, run errands, drive you to doctor's visits, or do other chores you feel too tired to do.

- **Eat a well-balanced diet.** Choose a diet that contains all the calories and protein your body needs. Calories will help keep your weight up, and extra protein can help repair tissues that have been harmed by cancer treatment. Talk to your doctor, nurse, or dietitian about the diet that is right for you. (To learn more, see Appetite Changes on page 18.)

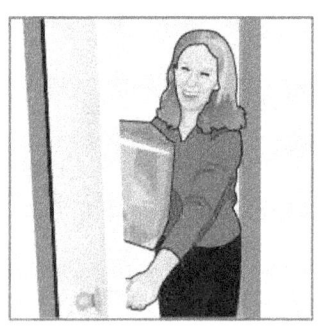

- **Stand up slowly.** You may feel dizzy if you stand up too fast. When you get up from lying down, sit for a minute before you stand.

When you get up from lying down, sit for a moment before you stand.

Your doctor or nurse will check your blood cell count throughout your chemotherapy. You may need a blood transfusion if your red blood cell count falls too low. Your doctor may also prescribe a medicine to boost (speed up) the growth of red blood cells or suggest that you take iron or other vitamins.

Call your doctor or nurse if:

- Your level of fatigue changes or you are not able to do your usual activities

- You feel dizzy or like you are going to faint

- You feel short of breath

- It feels like your heart is pounding or beating very fast

For more information on how to manage fatigue that may be caused by anemia, see page 26.

Appetite Changes

What they are and why they occur

Chemotherapy can cause appetite changes. You may lose your appetite because of nausea (feeling like you are going to throw up), mouth and throat problems that make it painful to eat, or drugs that cause you to lose your taste for food. The changes can also come from feeling depressed or tired. Appetite loss may last for a day, a few weeks, or even months.

It is important to eat well, even when you have no appetite. This means eating and drinking foods that have plenty of protein, vitamins, and calories. Eating well helps your body fight infection and repair tissues that are damaged by chemotherapy. Not eating well can lead to weight loss, weakness, and fatigue.

Some cancer treatments cause weight gain or an increase in your appetite. Be sure to ask your doctor, nurse, or dietitian what types of appetite changes you might expect and how to manage them.

Ways to manage

- Eat 5 to 6 small meals or snacks each day instead of 3 big meals. Choose foods and drinks that are high in calories and protein. See page 54 for a list of these foods.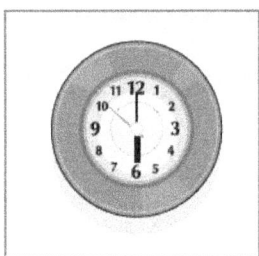

- Set a daily schedule for eating your meals and snacks. Eat when it is time to eat, rather than when you feel hungry. You may not feel hungry while you are on chemotherapy, but you still need to eat.

- Drink milkshakes, smoothies, juice, or soup if you do not feel like eating solid foods. Liquids like these can help provide the protein, vitamins, and calories your body needs. See page 53 for a list of liquid foods.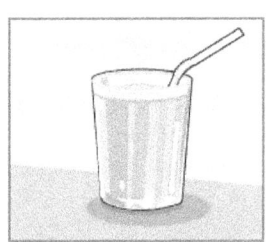

- Use plastic forks and spoons. Some types of chemo give you a metal taste in your mouth. Eating with plastic can help decrease the metal taste. Cooking in glass pots and pans can also help.

■ Increase your appetite by doing something active. For instance, you might have more of an appetite if you take a short walk before lunch. Also, be careful not to decrease your appetite by drinking too much liquid before or during meals.

■ Change your routine. This may mean eating in a different place, such as the dining room rather than the kitchen. It can also mean eating with other people instead of eating alone. If you eat alone, you may want to listen to the radio or watch TV. You may also want to vary your diet by trying new foods and recipes.

■ Talk with your doctor, nurse, or dietitian. He or she may want you to take extra vitamins or nutrition supplements (such as high protein drinks). If you cannot eat for a long time and are losing weight, you may need to take drugs that increase your appetite or receive nutrition through an IV or feeding tube.

NCI's book "Eating Hints: Before, During, and After Cancer Treatment" provides more tips for making eating easier. You can get a free copy at www.cancer.gov/publications or 1-800-4-CANCER (1-800-422-6237).

Bleeding

What it is and why it occurs

Platelets are cells that make your blood clot when you bleed. Chemotherapy can lower the number of platelets because it affects your bone marrow's ability to make them. A low platelet count is called **thrombocytopenia**. This condition may cause bruises (even when you have not been hit or have not bumped into anything), bleeding from your nose or in your mouth, or a rash of tiny, red dots.

Ways to manage

Do:

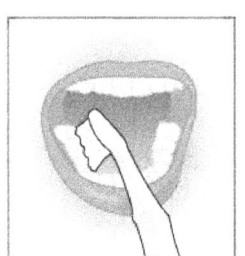

- Brush your teeth with a very soft toothbrush
- Soften the bristles of your toothbrush by running hot water over them before you brush
- Blow your nose gently

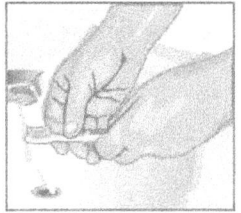

- Be careful when using scissors, knives, or other sharp objects
- Use an electric shaver instead of a razor
- Apply gentle but firm pressure to any cuts you get until the bleeding stops
- Wear shoes all the time, even inside the house or hospital

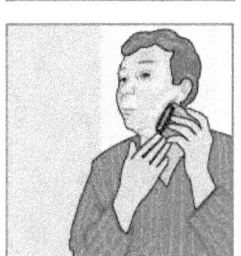

Do <u>not</u>:

- Use dental floss or toothpicks
- Play sports or do other activities during which you could get hurt
- Use tampons, enemas, suppositories, or rectal thermometers
- Wear clothes with tight collars, wrists, or waistbands

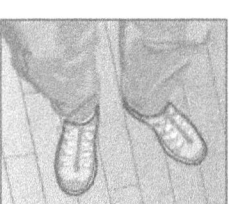

Check with your doctor or nurse before:

- Drinking beer, wine, or other types of alcohol
- Having sex
- Taking vitamins, herbs, minerals, dietary supplements, aspirin, or other over-the-counter medicines. Some of these products can change how chemotherapy works.

Check with your doctor or nurse before taking any vitamins, herbs, minerals, dietary supplements, aspirin, or other over-the-counter medicines.

Let your doctor know if you are constipated.

He or she may prescribe a stool softener to prevent straining and rectal bleeding when you go to the bathroom. For more information on **constipation**, see page 22.

Your doctor or nurse will check your platelet count often.

You may need medication, a platelet transfusion, or a delay in your chemotherapy treatment if your platelet count is too low.

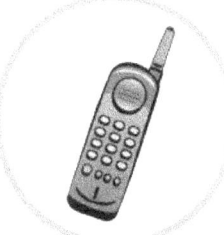

Call your doctor or nurse if you have any of these symptoms:

- Bruises, especially if you did not bump into anything
- Small, red spots on your skin
- Red- or pink-colored urine
- Black or bloody bowel movements
- Bleeding from your gums or nose
- Heavy bleeding during your menstrual period or for a prolonged period
- Vaginal bleeding not caused by your period
- Headaches or changes in your vision
- A warm or hot feeling in your arm or leg
- Feeling very sleepy or confused

Constipation

What it is and why it occurs

Constipation is when bowel movements become less frequent and stools are hard, dry, and difficult to pass. You may have painful bowel movements and feel bloated or nauseous. You may belch, pass a lot of gas, and have stomach cramps or pressure in the rectum.

Drugs such as chemotherapy and pain medicine can cause constipation. It can also happen when people are not active and spend a lot of time sitting or lying down. Constipation can also be due to eating foods that are low in fiber or not drinking enough fluids.

Ways to manage

- Keep a record of your bowel movements. Show this record to your doctor or nurse and talk about what is normal for you. This makes it easier to figure out whether you have constipation.

- Drink at least 8 cups of water or other fluids each day. Many people find that drinking warm or hot fluids, such as coffee and tea, helps with constipation. Fruit juices, such as prune juice, may also be helpful.

When you eat more fiber, be sure to drink more fluids.

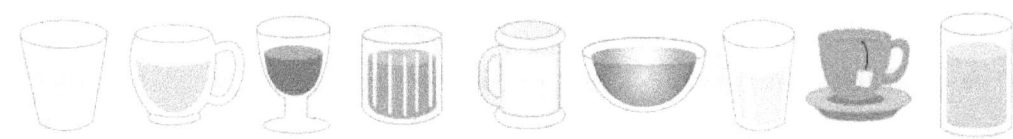

- Be active every day. You can be active by walking, riding a bike, or doing yoga. If you cannot walk, ask about exercises that you can do in a chair or bed. Talk with your doctor or nurse about ways you can be more active.

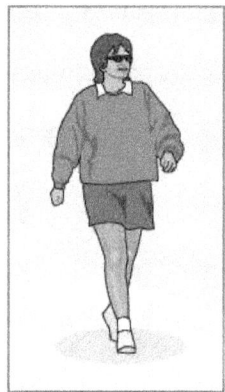

Check with your doctor or nurse before using fiber supplements, laxatives, stool softeners, or enemas.

■ **Ask your doctor, nurse, or dietitian about foods that are high in fiber.** Eating high-fiber foods and drinking lots of fluids can help soften your stools. Good sources of fiber include whole-grain breads and cereals, dried beans and peas, raw vegetables, fresh and dried fruit, nuts, seeds, and popcorn. (To learn more, see the list of high-fiber foods on page 55.)

■ **Let your doctor or nurse know if you have not had a bowel movement in 2 days.** Your doctor may suggest a fiber supplement, laxative, stool softener, or enema. Do not use these treatments without first checking with your doctor or nurse.

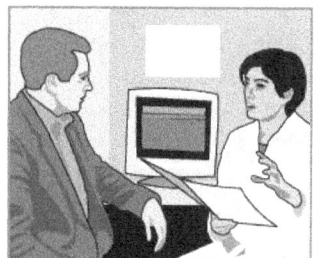

Diarrhea

What it is and why it occurs

Diarrhea is frequent bowel movements that may be soft, loose, or watery. Chemotherapy can cause diarrhea because it harms healthy cells that line your large and small intestines. It may also speed up your bowels. Diarrhea can also be caused by infections or drugs used to treat constipation.

Ways to manage

- Eat 5 or 6 small meals and snacks each day instead of 3 large meals.

- Ask your doctor or nurse about foods that are high in salts such as sodium and potassium. Your body can lose these salts when you have diarrhea, and it is important to replace them. Foods that are high in sodium or potassium include bananas, oranges, peach and apricot nectar, and boiled or mashed potatoes.

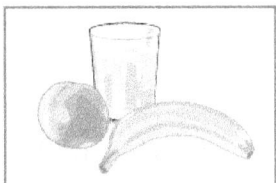

- Drink 8 to 12 cups of clear liquids each day. These include water, clear broth, ginger ale, or sports drinks such as Gatorade® or Propel®. Drink slowly, and choose drinks that are at room temperature. Let carbonated drinks lose their fizz before you drink them. Add extra water if drinks make you thirsty or nauseous (feeling like you are going to throw up).

- Eat low-fiber foods. Foods that are high in fiber can make diarrhea worse. Low-fiber foods include bananas, white rice, white toast, and plain or vanilla yogurt. See page 56 for other low-fiber foods.

- Let your doctor or nurse know if your diarrhea lasts for more than 24 hours or if you have pain and cramping along with diarrhea. Your doctor may prescribe a medicine to control the diarrhea. You may also need IV fluids to replace the water and nutrients you lost. Do not take any medicine for diarrhea without first asking your doctor or nurse.

Ask your doctor or nurse before taking medicine for diarrhea.

- Be gentle when you wipe yourself after a bowel movement. Instead of toilet paper, use a baby wipe or squirt of water from a spray bottle to clean yourself after bowel movements. Let your doctor or nurse know if your rectal area is sore or bleeds or if you have hemorrhoids.

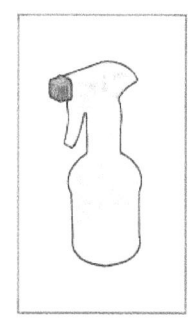

- Ask your doctor if you should try a clear liquid diet. This can give your bowels time to rest. Most people stay on this type of diet for 5 days or less. See page 52 for a list of clear liquids.

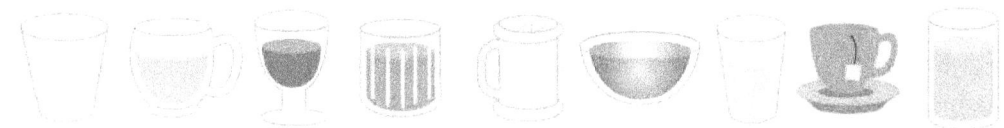

Stay away from:

- Drinks that are very hot or very cold

- Beer, wine, and other types of alcohol

- Milk or milk products, such as ice cream, milkshakes, sour cream, and cheese

- Spicy foods, such as hot sauce, salsa, chili, and curry dishes

- Greasy and fried foods, such as french fries and hamburgers

- Foods or drinks with caffeine, such as regular coffee, black tea, cola, and chocolate

- Foods or drinks that cause gas, such as cooked dried beans, cabbage, broccoli, and soy milk and other soy products

- Foods that are high in fiber, such as cooked dried beans, raw fruits and vegetables, nuts, and whole-wheat breads and cereals

To learn more about ways to manage diarrhea during cancer treatment read *Eating Hints: Before, During, and After Cancer Treatment*, a book from NCI. You can get a free copy at www.cancer.gov/publications or by calling 1-800-4-CANCER (1-800-422-6237).

Fatigue

What it is and why it occurs

Fatigue from chemotherapy can range from a mild to extreme feeling of being tired. Many people describe fatigue as feeling weak, weary, worn out, heavy, or slow. Resting does not always help.

Many people say they feel fatigue during chemotherapy and even for weeks or months after treatment is over. Fatigue can be caused by the type of chemotherapy, the effort of making frequent visits to the doctor, or feelings such as stress, anxiety, and depression. If you receive radiation therapy along with chemotherapy, your fatigue may be more severe.

Fatigue can also be caused by:

- Anemia (see page 16)
- Pain (see page 42)
- Medications
- Appetite changes (see page 18)
- Trouble sleeping
- Lack of activity
- Trouble breathing
- Infection (see page 30)
- Doing too much at one time
- Other medical problems

Fatigue can happen all at once or little by little. People feel fatigue in different ways. You may feel more or less fatigue than someone else who gets the same type of chemotherapy.

Ways to manage

- **Relax.** You might want to try meditation, prayer, yoga, guided imagery, visualization, or other ways to relax and decrease stress.

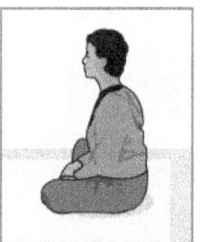

- **Eat and drink well.** Often, this means 5 to 6 small meals and snacks rather than 3 large meals. Keep foods around that are easy to fix, such as canned soups, frozen meals, yogurt, and cottage cheese. Drink plenty of fluids each day—about 8 cups of water or juice.

- **Plan time to rest.** You may feel better when you rest or take a short nap during the day. Many people say that it helps to rest for just 10 to 15 minutes rather than nap for a long time. If you nap, try to sleep for less than 1 hour. Keeping naps short will help you sleep better at night.

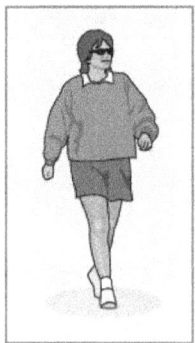

- **Be active.** Research shows that exercise can ease fatigue and help you sleep better at night. Try going for a 15-minute walk, doing yoga, or riding an exercise bike. Plan to be active when you have the most energy. Talk with your doctor or nurse about ways you can be active while getting chemotherapy.

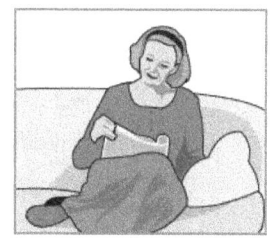

- **Try not to do too much.** With fatigue, you may not have enough energy to do all the things you want to do. Choose the activities you want to do and let someone else help with the others. Try quiet activities, such as reading, knitting, or learning a new language on tape.

- **Sleep at least 8 hours each night.** This may be more sleep than you needed before chemotherapy. You are likely to sleep better at night when you are active during the day. You may also find it helpful to relax before going to bed. For instance, you might read a book, work on a jigsaw puzzle, listen to music, or do other quiet hobbies.

- **Plan a work schedule that works for you.** Fatigue may affect the amount of energy you have for your job. You may feel well enough to work your full schedule. Or you may need to work less—maybe just a few hours a day or a few days each week. If your job allows, you may want to talk with your boss about ways to work from home. Or you may want to go on medical leave (stop working for a while) while getting chemotherapy.

- **Let others help.** Ask family members and friends to help when you feel fatigue. Perhaps they can help with household chores or drive you to and from doctor's visits. They might also help by shopping for food and cooking meals for you to eat now or freeze for later.

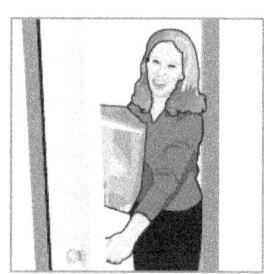

- **Learn from others who have cancer.** People who have cancer can help by sharing ways that they manage fatigue. One way to meet others is by joining a support group—either in person or online. Talk with your doctor or nurse to learn more.

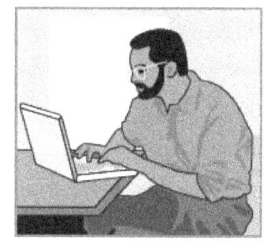

- **Keep a diary of how you feel each day.** This will help you plan how to best use your time. Share your diary with your nurse. Let your doctor or nurse know if you notice changes in your energy level, whether you have lots of energy or are very tired.

- **Talk with your doctor or nurse.** Your doctor may prescribe medication that can help decrease fatigue, give you a sense of well-being, and increase your appetite. He or she may also suggest treatment if your fatigue is from anemia. (To learn more about anemia, see page 16.)

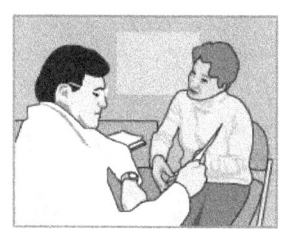

Hair Loss

What it is and why it occurs

Hair loss (also called **alopecia**) is when some or all of your hair falls out. This can happen anywhere on your body: your head, face, arms, legs, underarms, or the pubic area between your legs. Many people are upset by the loss of their hair and find it the most difficult part of chemotherapy.

Some types of chemotherapy damage the cells that cause hair growth. Hair loss often starts 2 to 3 weeks after chemotherapy begins. Your scalp may hurt at first. Then you may lose your hair, either a little at a time or in clumps. It takes about 1 week for all your hair to fall out. Almost always, your hair will grow back 2 to 3 months after chemotherapy is over. You may notice that your hair starts growing back even while you are getting chemotherapy.

Your hair will be very fine when it starts growing back. Also, your new hair may not look or feel the same as it did before. For instance, your hair may be thin instead of thick, curly instead of straight, and darker or lighter in color.

Hair often grows back 2 to 3 months after chemotherapy is over.

Ways to manage

Before hair loss:

- **Talk with your doctor or nurse.** He or she will know if you are likely to have hair loss.

- **Cut your hair short or shave your head.** You might feel more in control of hair loss if you first cut your hair or shave your head. This often makes hair loss easier to manage. If you shave your head, use an electric shaver instead of a razor.

If you plan to buy a wig, do so while you still have hair.

- **The best time to choose your wig is before chemotherapy starts.** This way, you can match the wig to the color and style of your hair. You might also take it to your hair dresser who can style the wig to look like your own hair. Make sure to choose a wig that feels comfortable and does not hurt your scalp.

- **Ask if your insurance company will pay for a wig.** If it will not, you can deduct the cost of your wig as a medical expense on your income tax. Some groups also have free "wig banks." Your doctor, nurse, or social worker will know if there is a wig bank near you.

- **Be gentle when you wash your hair.** Use a mild shampoo, such as a baby shampoo. Dry your hair by patting (not rubbing) it with a soft towel.

- **Do not use items that can hurt your scalp.** These include:
  - Straightening or curling irons
  - Brush rollers or curlers
  - Electric hair dryers
  - Hair bands and clips
  - Hairsprays
  - Hair dyes
  - Products to perm or relax your hair

After hair loss:

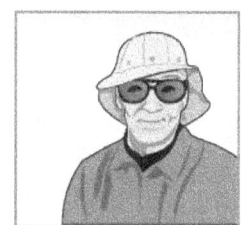

- **Protect your scalp.** Your scalp may hurt during and after hair loss. Protect it by wearing a hat, turban, or scarf when you are outside. Try to avoid places that are very hot or very cold. This includes tanning beds and outside in the sun or cold air. And always apply sunscreen or sunblock to protect your scalp.

- **Stay warm.** You may feel colder once you lose your hair. Wear a hat, turban, scarf, or wig to help you stay warm.

- **Sleep on a satin pillow case.** Satin creates less friction than cotton when you sleep on it. Therefore, you may find satin pillow cases more comfortable.

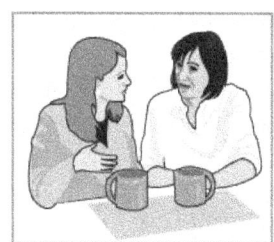

- **Talk about your feelings.** Many people feel angry, depressed, or embarrassed about hair loss. If you are very worried or upset, you might want to talk about these feelings with a doctor, nurse, family member, close friend, or someone who has had hair loss caused by cancer treatment.

Ways to learn more

American Cancer Society
Offers a variety of services to people with cancer and their families, including referrals to low-cost wig banks.

Call: 1-800-ACS-2345 (1-800-227-2345)

TTY: 1-866-228-4327

Visit: www.cancer.org

Infection

What it is and why it occurs

Some types of chemotherapy make it harder for your bone marrow to produce new **white blood cells**. White blood cells help your body fight infection. Therefore, it is important to avoid infections, since chemotherapy decreases the number of your white blood cells.

There are many types of white blood cells. One type is called **neutrophil**. When your neutrophil count is low, it is called **neutropenia**. Your doctor or nurse may do blood tests to find out whether you have neutropenia.

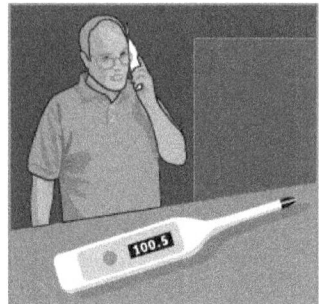

It is important to watch for signs of infection when you have neutropenia. Check for fever at least once a day, or as often as your doctor or nurse tells you to. You may find it best to use a digital thermometer. Call your doctor or nurse if your temperature is 100.5°F or higher.

Call your doctor or nurse right away if you have a fever of 100.5°F or higher.

Ways to manage

■ **Your doctor or nurse will check your white blood cell count throughout your treatment.** If chemotherapy is likely to make your white blood cell count very low, you may get medicine to raise your white blood cell count and lower your risk of infection.

■ **Wash your hands often with soap and water.** Be sure to wash your hands before cooking and eating, and after you use the bathroom, blow your nose, cough, sneeze, or touch animals. Carry hand sanitizer for times when you are not near soap and water.

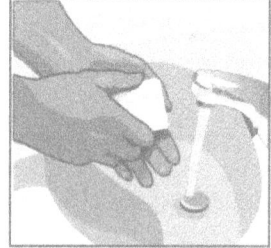

■ **Use sanitizing wipes to clean surfaces and items that you touch.** This includes public telephones, ATM machines, doorknobs, and other common items.

■ **Be gentle and thorough when you wipe yourself after a bowel movement.** Instead of toilet paper, use a baby wipe or squirt of water from a spray bottle to clean yourself. Let your doctor or nurse know if your rectal area is sore or bleeds or if you have hemorrhoids.

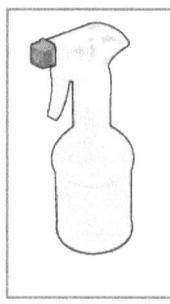

- **Stay away from people who are sick.** This includes people with colds, flu, measles, or chicken pox. You also need to stay away from children who just had a "live virus" vaccine for chicken pox or polio. Call your doctor, nurse, or local health department if you have any questions.

- **Stay away from crowds.** Try not to be around a lot of people. For instance, plan to go shopping or to the movies when the stores and theaters are less crowded.

- **Be careful not to cut or nick yourself.** Do not cut or tear your nail cuticles. Use an electric shaver instead of a razor. And be extra careful when using scissors, needles, or knives.

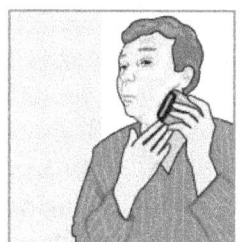

- **Watch for signs of infection around your catheter.** Signs include drainage, redness, swelling, or soreness. Let your doctor or nurse know about any changes you notice near your catheter.

- **Maintain good mouth care.** Brush your teeth after meals and before you go to bed. Use a very soft toothbrush. You can make the bristles even softer by running hot water over them just before you brush. Use a mouth rinse that does not contain alcohol. Check with your doctor or nurse before going to the dentist. (For more about taking care of your mouth, see page 35.)

- **Take good care of your skin.** Do not squeeze or scratch pimples. Use lotion to soften and heal dry, cracked skin. Dry yourself after a bath or shower by gently patting (not rubbing) your skin. (For more information about taking care of your skin, see page 47.)

- **Clean cuts right away.** Use warm water, soap, and an antiseptic to clean your cuts. Do this every day until your cut has a scab over it.

- **Be careful around animals.** Do not clean your cat's litter box, pick up dog waste, or clean bird cages or fish tanks. Be sure to wash your hands after touching pets and other animals.

- **Do not get a flu shot or other type of vaccine without first asking your doctor or nurse.** Some vaccines contain a live virus, which you should not be exposed to.

- **Keep hot foods hot and cold foods cold.** Do not leave leftovers sitting out. Put them in the refrigerator as soon as you are done eating.

- **Wash raw vegetables and fruits well before eating them.**

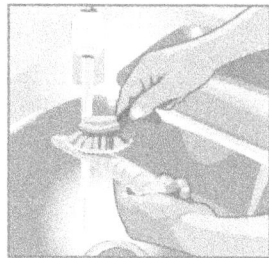

- **Do not eat raw or undercooked fish, seafood, meat, chicken, or eggs.** These may have bacteria that can cause infection.

- **Do not have food or drinks that are moldy, spoiled, or past the freshness date.**

Do not take drugs that reduce fever without first talking with your doctor or nurse.

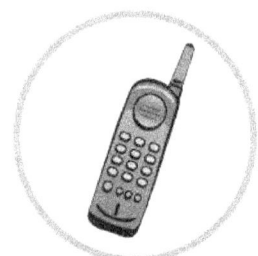

■ **Call your doctor right away (even on the weekend or in the middle of the night) if you think you have an infection.** Be sure you know how to reach your doctor after office hours and on weekends. Call if you have a fever of 100.5°F or higher, or when you have chills or sweats. Do not take aspirin, acetaminophen (such as Tylenol®), ibuprofen products, or any other drugs that reduce fever without first talking with your doctor or nurse. Other signs of infection include:

- Redness
- Swelling
- Rash
- Chills
- Cough
- Earache

- Headache
- Stiff neck
- Bloody or cloudy urine
- Painful or frequent need to urinate
- Sinus pain or pressure

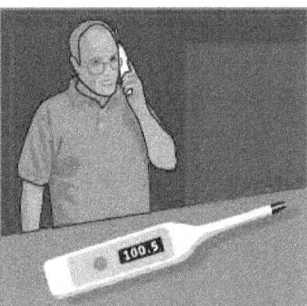

Be sure you know how to reach your doctor or nurse after office hours and on weekends.

Write the number to call in an emergency here:

Infertility

What it is and why it occurs

Some types of chemotherapy can cause **infertility**. For a woman, this means that you may not be able to get pregnant. For a man, this means you may not be able to get a woman pregnant.

In women, chemotherapy may damage the ovaries. This damage can lower the number of healthy eggs in the ovaries. It can also lower the **hormones** produced by them. The drop in hormones can lead to early menopause. Early menopause and fewer healthy eggs can cause infertility.

In men, chemotherapy may damage sperm cells, which grow and divide quickly. Infertility may occur because chemotherapy can lower the number of sperm, make sperm less able to move, or cause other types of damage.

Whether or not you become infertile depends on the type of chemotherapy you get, your age, and whether you have other health problems. Infertility can last the rest of your life.

Before treatment starts, tell your doctor or nurse if you want to have children in the future.

Ways to manage

For WOMEN, talk with your doctor or nurse about:

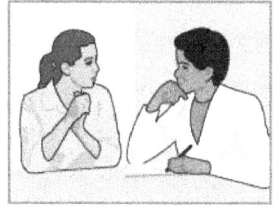

- **Whether you want to have children.** Before you start chemotherapy, let your doctor or nurse know if you might want to get pregnant in the future. He or she may talk with you about ways to preserve your eggs to use after treatment ends or refer you to a fertility specialist.

- **Birth control.** It is very important that you do not get pregnant while getting chemotherapy. These drugs can hurt the fetus, especially in the first 3 months of pregnancy. If you have not yet gone through menopause, talk with your doctor or nurse about birth control and ways to keep from getting pregnant.

- **Pregnancy.** If you still have menstrual periods, your doctor or nurse may ask you to have a pregnancy test before you start chemotherapy. If you are pregnant, your doctor or nurse will talk with you about other treatment options.

Chemotherapy can cause birth defects. Do not get pregnant while you are getting treatment.

Talk with your doctor or nurse about saving your sperm before you start treatment, if you want to father children in the future.

For MEN, talk with your doctor or nurse about:

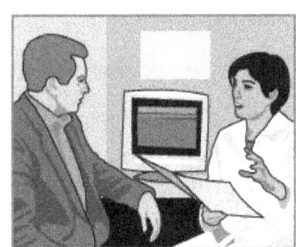

- **Whether you want to have children.** Before you start chemotherapy, let your doctor or nurse know if you might want to father children in the future. He or she may talk with you about ways to preserve your sperm to use in the future or refer you to a fertility specialist.

- **Birth control.** It is very important that your spouse or partner does not get pregnant while you are getting chemotherapy. Chemotherapy can damage your sperm and cause birth defects.

Chemotherapy may damage sperm and cause birth defects. Make sure that your spouse or partner does not get pregnant while you are in treatment.

Ways to learn more

American Cancer Society
Offers a variety of services to people with cancer and their families.

Call:	1-800-ACS-2345 (1-800-227-2345)
TTY:	1-866-228-4327
Visit:	www.cancer.org

fertileHOPE
A LIVESTRONG initiative dedicated to providing reproductive information, support, and hope to cancer patients and survivors whose medical treatments present the risk of infertility.

Call:	1-866-965-7205
Visit:	www.fertilehope.org

Mouth and Throat Changes

What they are and why they occur

Some types of chemotherapy harm fast-growing cells, such as those that line your mouth, throat, and lips. This can affect your teeth, gums, the lining of your mouth, and the glands that make saliva. Most mouth problems go away a few days after chemotherapy is over.

Mouth and throat problems may include:

- Dry mouth (having little or no saliva)

- Changes in taste and smell (such as when food tastes like metal or chalk, has no taste, or does not taste or smell like it used to)

- Infections of your gums, teeth, or tongue

- Increased sensitivity to hot or cold foods

- Mouth sores

- Trouble eating when your mouth gets very sore

Ways to manage

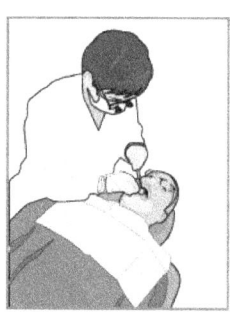

- Visit a dentist at least 2 weeks before starting chemotherapy. It is important to have your mouth as healthy as possible. This means getting all your dental work done before chemotherapy starts. If you cannot go to the dentist before chemotherapy starts, ask your doctor or nurse when it is safe to go. Be sure to tell your dentist that you have cancer and about your treatment plan.

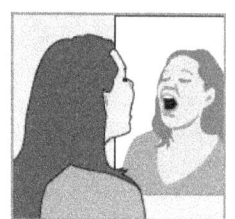

- Check your mouth and tongue every day. This way, you can see or feel problems (such as mouth sores, white spots, or infections) as soon as they start. Inform your doctor or nurse about these problems right away.

Visit your dentist at least 2 weeks before starting chemotherapy.

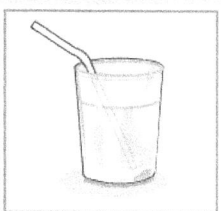

- Keep your mouth moist. You can keep your mouth moist by sipping water throughout the day, sucking on ice chips or sugar-free hard candy, or chewing sugar-free gum. Ask your doctor or nurse about saliva substitutes if your mouth is always dry.

■ Clean your mouth, teeth, gums, and tongue.

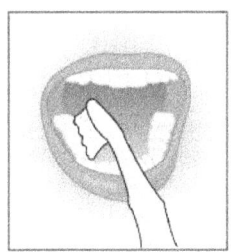

- Brush your teeth, gums, and tongue after each meal and at bedtime.

- Use an extra-soft toothbrush. You can make the bristles even softer by rinsing your toothbrush in hot water before you brush.

- If brushing is painful, try cleaning your teeth with cotton swabs or Toothettes®.

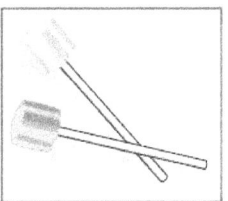

- Use a fluoride toothpaste or special fluoride gel that your dentist prescribes.

- Do not use mouthwash that has alcohol. Instead, rinse your mouth 3 to 4 times a day with a solution of 1/4 teaspoon baking soda and 1/8 teaspoon salt in 1 cup of warm water. Follow this with a plain water rinse.

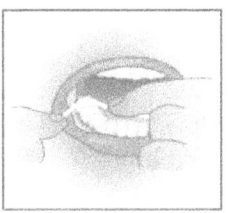

- Gently floss your teeth every day. If your gums bleed or hurt, avoid those areas but floss your other teeth. Ask your doctor or nurse about flossing if your platelet count is low. (See the section called "Bleeding" on page 20 for more information on platelets.)

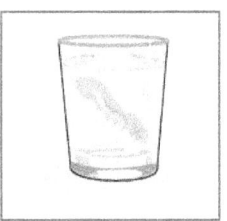

- If you wear dentures, make sure they fit well and keep them clean. Also, limit the length of time that you wear them.

■ Be careful what you eat when your mouth is sore.

- Choose foods that are moist, soft, and easy to chew or swallow. These include cooked cereals, mashed potatoes, and scrambled eggs.

- Use a blender to puree cooked foods so that they are easier to eat. To help avoid infection, be sure to wash all blender parts before and after using them. If possible, it is best to wash them in a dishwasher.

- Take small bites of food, chew slowly, and sip liquids while you eat.

- Soften food with gravy, sauces, broth, yogurt, or other liquids.

- Eat foods that are cool or at room temperature. You may find that warm and hot foods hurt your mouth or throat.

- Suck on ice chips or popsicles. These can relieve mouth pain.

- Ask your dietitian for ideas of foods that are easy to eat. For ideas of soft foods that are easy on a sore mouth, see page 57.

Call your doctor, nurse, or dentist if your mouth hurts a lot. Your doctor or dentist may prescribe medicine for pain or to keep your mouth moist. Make sure to give your dentist the phone number of your doctor and nurse.

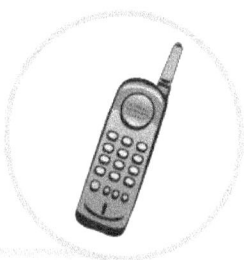

■ Stay away from things that can hurt, scrape, or burn your mouth, such as:

- Sharp or crunchy foods, such as crackers and potato or corn chips

- Spicy foods, such as hot sauce, curry dishes, salsa, and chili

- Citrus fruits or juices such as orange, lemon, and grapefruit

- Food and drinks that have a lot of sugar, such as candy or soda

- Beer, wine, and other types of alcohol

- Toothpicks or other sharp objects

- Tobacco products, including cigarettes, pipes, cigars, and chewing tobacco

Do not use tobacco or drink alcohol if your mouth is sore.

Ways to learn more

National Oral Health Information Clearinghouse
A service of the National Institutes of Dental and Craniofacial Research that provides oral health information for special care patients.

Call: 1-866-232-4528

Visit: www.nidcr.nih.gov

E-mail: nidcrinfo@mail.nih.gov

Smokefree.gov
Provides resources including information on quitlines, a step-by-step cessation guide, and publications to help you or someone you care about quit smoking.

Call: 1-877-44U-QUIT (1-877-448-7848)

Visit: www.smokefree.gov

Nausea and Vomiting

What they are and why they occur

Some types of chemotherapy can cause nausea, vomiting, or both. Nausea is when you feel sick to your stomach, like you are going to throw up. Vomiting is when you throw up. You may also have **dry heaves**, which is when your body tries to vomit even though your stomach is empty.

Nausea and vomiting can occur while you are getting chemotherapy, right after, or many hours or days later. You will most likely feel better on the days you do not get chemotherapy.

New drugs can help prevent nausea and vomiting. These are called **antiemetic** or **antinausea** drugs. You may need to take these drugs 1 hour before each chemotherapy treatment and for a few days after. How long you take them after chemotherapy will depend on the type of chemotherapy you are getting and how you react to it. If one antinausea drug does not work well for you, your doctor can prescribe a different one. You may need to take more than one type of drug to help with nausea. **Acupuncture** may also help. Talk with your doctor or nurse about treatments to control nausea and vomiting caused by chemotherapy.

Ways to manage

- **Prevent nausea.** One way to prevent vomiting is to prevent nausea. Try having bland, easy-to-digest foods and drinks that do not upset your stomach. These include plain crackers, toast, and gelatin. To learn more, see the list of foods and drinks that are easy on the stomach on page 58.

- **Plan when it's best for you to eat and drink.** Some people feel better when they eat a light meal or snack before chemotherapy. Others feel better when they have chemotherapy on an empty stomach (nothing to eat or drink for 2 to 3 hours before treatment). After treatment, wait at least 1 hour before you eat or drink.

- **Eat small meals and snacks.** Instead of 3 large meals each day, you might feel better if you eat 5 or 6 small meals and snacks. Do not drink a lot before or during meals. Also, do not lie down right after you eat.

- **Have foods and drinks that are warm or cool (not hot or cold).** Give hot foods and drinks time to cool down, or make them colder by adding ice. You can warm up cold foods by taking them out of the refrigerator 1 hour before you eat or warming them slightly in a microwave. Drink cola or ginger ale that is warm and has lost its fizz.

Eat 5 or 6 small meals and snacks each day instead of 3 large ones.

- Stay away from foods and drinks with strong smells. These include coffee, fish, onions, garlic, and foods that are cooking.

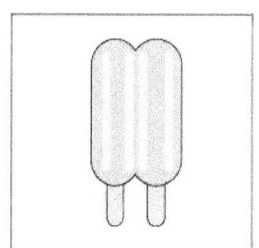

- Try small bites of popsicles or fruit ices. You may also find sucking on ice chips helpful.

- Suck on sugar-free mints or tart candies. But do not use tart candies if you have mouth or throat sores.

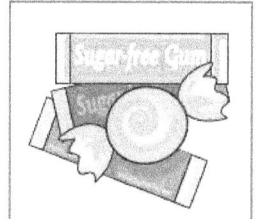

- Relax before treatment. You may feel less nausea if you relax before each chemotherapy treatment. Meditate, do deep breathing exercises, or imagine scenes or experiences that make you feel peaceful. You can also do quiet hobbies such as reading, listening to music, or knitting.

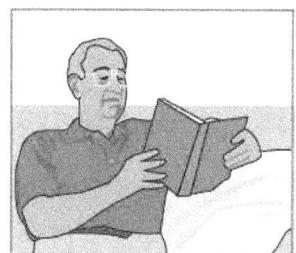

- When you feel like vomiting, breathe deeply and slowly or get fresh air. You might also distract yourself by chatting with friends or family, listening to music, or watching a movie or TV.

- Talk with your doctor or nurse. Your doctor can give you drugs to help prevent nausea during and after chemotherapy. Be sure to take these drugs as ordered and let your doctor or nurse know if they do not work. You might also ask your doctor or nurse about acupuncture, which can help relieve nausea and vomiting caused by cancer treatment.

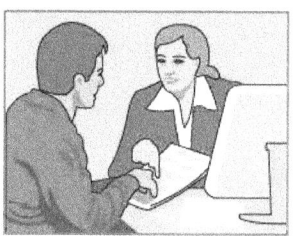

Tell your doctor or nurse if you vomit for more than 1 day or right after you drink.

Let your doctor or nurse know if your medicine for nausea is not working.

To learn more about dealing with nausea and vomiting during cancer treatment read *Eating Hints: Before, During, and After Cancer Treatment*, a book from NCI. You can get a free copy at www.cancer.gov/publications or by calling 1-800-4-CANCER (1-800-422-6237).

Nervous System Changes

What they are and why they occur

Chemotherapy can cause damage to your nervous system. Many nervous system problems get better within a year of when you finish chemotherapy, but some may last the rest of your life. Symptoms may include:

- Tingling, burning, weakness, or numbness in your hands or feet

- Feeling colder than normal

- Pain when walking

- Weak, sore, tired, or achy muscles

- Being clumsy and losing your balance

- Trouble picking up objects or buttoning your clothes

- Shaking or trembling

- Hearing loss

- Stomach pain, such as constipation or heartburn

- Fatigue

- Confusion and memory problems

- Dizziness

- Depression

Let your doctor or nurse know right away if you notice any nervous system changes. It is important to treat these problems as soon as possible.

Ways to manage

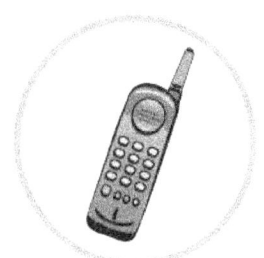

- Let your doctor or nurse know right away if you notice any nervous system changes. It is important to treat these problems as soon as possible.

- Be careful when handling knives, scissors, and other sharp or dangerous objects.

- Avoid falling. Walk slowly, hold onto handrails when using the stairs, and put no-slip bath mats in your bathtub or shower. Make sure there are no area rugs or cords to trip over.

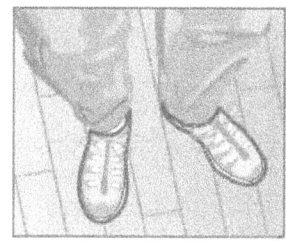

- Always wear sneakers, tennis shoes, or other footwear with rubber soles.

- Check the temperature of your bath water with a thermometer. This will keep you from getting burned by water that is too hot.

- Be extra careful to avoid burning or cutting yourself while cooking.

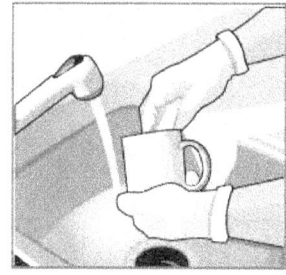

- Wear gloves when working in the garden, cooking, or washing dishes.

- Rest when you need to.

- Steady yourself when you walk by using a cane or other device.

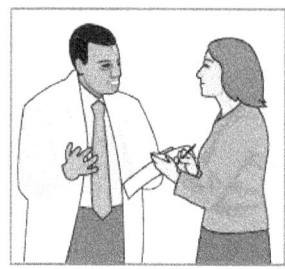

- Talk to your doctor or nurse if you notice memory problems, feel confused, or are depressed.

- Ask your doctor for pain medicine if you need it.

Pain

What it is and why it occurs

Some types of chemotherapy cause painful side effects. These include burning, numbness, and tingling or shooting pains in your hands and feet. Mouth sores, headaches, muscle pains, and stomach pains can also occur.

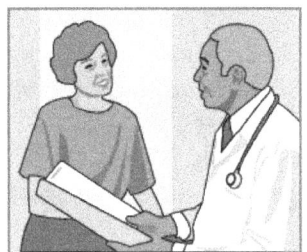

Pain can be caused by the cancer itself or by chemotherapy. Doctors and nurses have ways to decrease or relieve your pain.

Be sure to tell your doctor or nurse if you have pain.

Ways to manage

▓ Talk about your pain with a doctor, nurse, or pharmacist. Be specific and describe:

- Where you feel pain. Is it in one part of your body or all over?
- What the pain feels like. Is it sharp, dull, or throbbing? Does it come and go, or is it steady?
- How strong the pain is. Describe it on a scale of 0 to 10.
- How long the pain lasts. Does it last for a few minutes, an hour, or longer?
- What makes the pain better or worse. For instance, does an ice pack help? Or does the pain get worse if you move a certain way?
- Which medicines you take for pain. Do they help? How long do they last? How much do you take? How often?

▓ **Let your family and friends know about your pain.** They need to know about your pain so they can help you. If you are very tired or in a lot of pain, they can call your doctor or nurse for you. Knowing about your pain can also help them understand why you may be acting differently.

■ Practice pain control

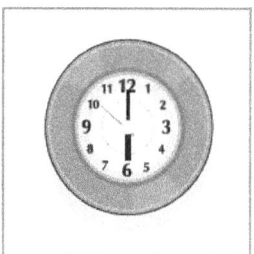

- Take your pain medicine on a regular schedule (by the clock) even when you are not in pain. This is very important when you have pain most of the time.

- Do not skip doses of your pain medicine. Pain is harder to control and manage if you wait until you are in a lot of pain before taking medicine.

- Try deep breathing, yoga, or other ways to relax. This can help reduce muscle tension, anxiety, and pain.

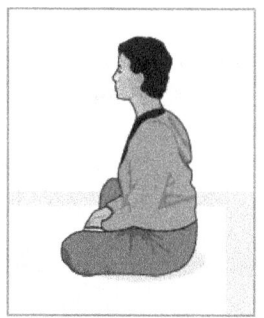

■ Ask to meet with a pain or palliative care specialist. This can be an oncologist, anesthesiologist, neurologist, neurosurgeon, nurse, or pharmacist who will talk with you about ways to control your pain.

■ Let your doctor, nurse, or pain specialist know if your pain changes. Your pain can change over the course of your treatment. When this happens, your pain medications may need to be changed.

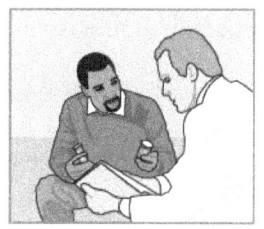

NCI's book, *Pain Control: Support for People With Cancer*, provides more tips about how to control pain from cancer and its treatment. You can get free copies at www.cancer.gov/publications or by calling 1-800-4-CANCER (1-800-422-6237).

Sexual Changes

What they are and why they occur

Some types of chemotherapy can cause sexual changes. These changes are different for women and men.

In women, chemotherapy may damage the ovaries, which can cause changes in hormone levels. Hormone changes can lead to problems like vaginal dryness and early menopause.

In men, chemotherapy can cause changes in hormone levels, decreased blood supply to the penis, or damage to the nerves that control the penis, all of which can lead to **impotence**.

Whether or not you have sexual changes during chemotherapy depends on if you have had these problems before, the type of chemotherapy you are getting, your age, and whether you have any other illnesses. Some problems, such as loss of interest in sex, are likely to improve once chemotherapy is over.

Problems for WOMEN include:

- Symptoms of menopause (for women not yet in menopause). These symptoms include:
  - Hot flashes
  - Vaginal dryness
  - Feeling irritable
  - Irregular or no menstrual periods

- Bladder or vaginal infections

- Vaginal discharge or itching

- Being too tired to have sex or not being interested in having sex

- Feeling too worried, stressed, or depressed to have sex

Problems for MEN include:

- Not being able to reach climax

- Impotence (not being able to get or keep an erection)

- Being too tired to have sex or not being interested in having sex

- Feeling too worried, stressed, or depressed to have sex

Ways to manage

For WOMEN:

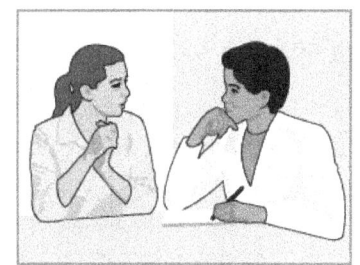

■ Talk with your doctor or nurse about:

- Sex. Ask your doctor or nurse if it is okay for you to have sex during chemotherapy. Most women can have sex, but it is a good idea to ask.

- Birth control. It is very important that you not get pregnant while having chemotherapy. Chemotherapy may hurt the fetus, especially in the first 3 months of pregnancy. If you have not yet gone through menopause, talk with your doctor or nurse about birth control and ways to keep from getting pregnant.

- Medications. Talk with your doctor, nurse, or pharmacist about medications that help with sexual problems. These include products to relieve vaginal dryness or a vaginal cream or suppository to reduce the chance of infection.

Talk with your doctor or nurse about ways to relieve vaginal dryness and prevent infection.

■ Wear cotton underwear (cotton underpants and pantyhose with cotton linings).

■ Do not wear tight pants or shorts.

■ Use a water-based vaginal lubricant (such as K-Y Jelly or Astroglide) when you have sex.

■ If sex is still painful because of dryness, ask your doctor or nurse about medications to help restore moisture in your vagina.

■ Cope with hot flashes by:

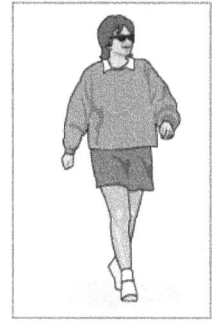

- Dressing in layers, with an extra sweater or jacket that you can take off.

- Being active. This includes walking, riding a bike, or other types of exercise.

- Reducing stress. Try yoga, meditation, or other ways to relax.

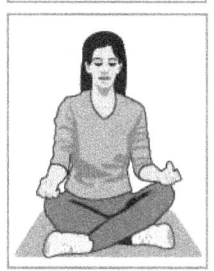

For MEN:

- **Talk with your doctor or nurse about:**

  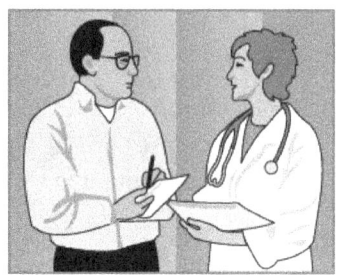

  - **Sex.** Ask your doctor or nurse if it is okay for you to have sex during chemotherapy. Most men can have sex, but it is a good idea to ask. Also, ask if you should use a condom when you have sex, since traces of chemotherapy may be in your semen.

  - **Birth control.** It is very important that your spouse or partner not get pregnant while you are getting chemotherapy. Chemotherapy can damage your sperm and cause birth defects.

If you are having sex less often, try activities that make you feel close to each other.

For men AND women:

- **Be open and honest with your spouse or partner.** Talk about your feelings and concerns.

- **Explore new ways to show love.** You and your spouse or partner may want to show your love for each other in new ways while you go through chemotherapy. For instance, if you are having sex less often, you may want to hug and cuddle more, bathe together, give each other massages, or try other activities that make you feel close to each other.

- **Talk with a doctor, nurse, social worker, or counselor.** If you and your spouse or partner are concerned about sexual problems, you may want to talk with someone who can help. This can be a psychiatrist, psychologist, social worker, marriage counselor, sex therapist, or clergy member.

Ways to learn more

American Cancer Society
Offers a variety of services to people with cancer and their families.

Call: 1-800-ACS-2345 (1-800-227-2345)

TTY: 1-866-228-4327

Visit: www.cancer.org

Skin and Nail Changes

What they are and why they occur

Some types of chemotherapy can damage the fast-growing cells in your skin and nails. While these changes may be painful and annoying, most are minor and do not require treatment. Many of them will get better once you have finished chemotherapy. However, major skin changes need to be treated right away because they can cause lifelong damage.

Minor skin changes may include:

- Itching, dryness, redness, rashes, and peeling

- Darker veins. Your veins may look darker when you get chemotherapy through an IV.

- Sensitivity to the sun (when you burn very quickly). This can happen even to people who have very dark skin color.

- Nail problems. This is when your nails become dark, turn yellow, or become brittle and cracked. Sometimes your nails will loosen and fall off, but new nails will grow back in.

Major skin changes need to be treated right away, because they can cause lifelong changes.

Major skin changes can be caused by:

- Radiation recall. Some chemotherapy causes skin in the area where you had radiation therapy to turn red (ranging from very light to bright red). Your skin may blister, peel, or be very painful.

- Chemotherapy leaking from your IV. You need to let your doctor or nurse know right away if you have burning or pain when you get IV chemotherapy.

- Allergic reactions to chemotherapy. Some skin changes mean that you are allergic to the chemotherapy. Let your doctor or nurse know right away if you have sudden and severe itching, rashes, or hives, along with wheezing or other trouble breathing.

Let your doctor or nurse know right away if you have burning or pain when you get IV chemotherapy.

Ways to manage

◼ Itching, dryness, redness, rashes, and peeling

- Apply cornstarch, as you would dusting powder.

- Take quick showers or sponge baths instead of long, hot baths.

- Pat (do not rub) yourself dry after bathing.

- Wash with a mild, moisturizing soap.

- Put on cream or lotion while your skin is still damp after washing. Tell your doctor or nurse if this does not help.

- Do not use perfume, cologne, or aftershave lotion that has alcohol.

- Take a colloidal oatmeal bath (special powder you add to bath water) when your whole body itches.

◼ Acne

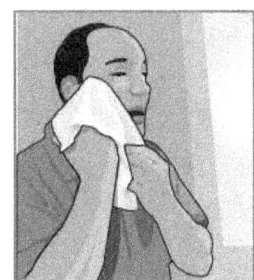

- Keep your face clean and dry.

- Ask your doctor or nurse if you can use medicated creams or soaps and which ones to use.

◼ Sensitivity to the sun

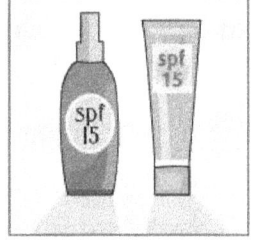

- Avoid direct sunlight. This means not being in the sun from 10 a.m. until 4 p.m. It is the time when the sun is strongest.

- Use sunscreen lotion with an SPF (skin protection factor) of 15 or higher. Or use ointments that block the sun's rays, such as those with zinc oxide.

- Keep your lips moist with a lip balm that has an SPF of 15 or higher.

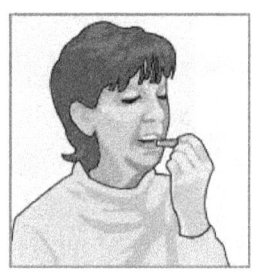

- Wear light-colored pants, long-sleeve cotton shirts, and hats with wide brims.

- Do not use tanning beds.

◼ Nail problems

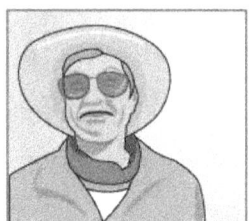

- Wear gloves when washing dishes, working in the garden, or cleaning the house.

- Use products to make your nails stronger. (Stop using these products if they hurt your nails or skin.)

- Let your doctor or nurse know if your cuticles are red and painful.

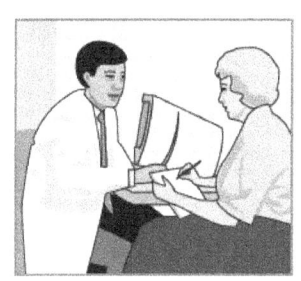

■ Radiation recall

- Protect the area of your skin that received radiation therapy from the sun.

- Do not use tanning beds.

- Place a cool, wet cloth where your skin hurts.

- Wear clothes that are made of cotton or other soft fabrics. This includes your underwear (bras, underpants, and t-shirts).

- Let your doctor or nurse know if you think you have radiation recall.

Urinary, Kidney, and Bladder Changes

What they are and why they occur

Some types of chemotherapy damage cells in the kidneys and bladder. Problems may include:

- Burning or pain when you begin to urinate or after you empty your bladder
- Frequent, more urgent need to urinate
- Not being able to urinate
- Not able to control the flow of urine from the bladder (**incontinence**)
- Blood in the urine
- Fever
- Chills
- Urine that is orange, red, green, or dark yellow or has a strong medicine odor

Some kidney and bladder problems will go away after you finish chemotherapy. Other problems can last for the rest of your life.

Drink plenty of fluids if you are getting chemotherapy that can damage the bladder and kidneys.

Ways to manage

- Your doctor or nurse will take urine and blood samples to check how well your bladder and kidneys are working.

- Drink plenty of fluids. Fluids will help flush the chemotherapy out of your bladder and kidneys. See the lists of clear liquids and liquid foods on pages 52 and 53.

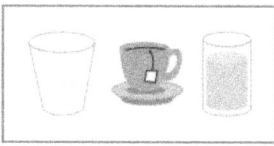

- Limit drinks that contain caffeine (such as black tea, coffee, and some cola products).

- Talk with your doctor or nurse if you have any of the problems listed above.

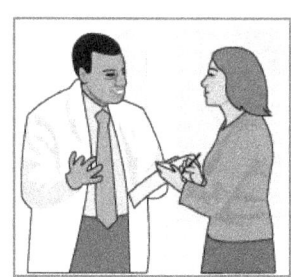

Other Side Effects

Flu-like symptoms

Some types of chemotherapy can make you feel like you have the flu. This is more likely to happen if you get chemotherapy along with biological therapy.

Flu-like symptoms may include:

- Muscle and joint aches
- Headache
- Fatigue
- Nausea
- Fever
- Chills
- Appetite loss

These symptoms may last from 1 to 3 days. An infection or the cancer itself can also cause them. Let your doctor or nurse know if you have any of these symptoms.

Fluid retention

Fluid retention is a buildup of fluid caused by chemotherapy, hormone changes caused by treatment, or your cancer. It can cause your face, hands, feet, or stomach to feel swollen and puffy. Sometimes fluid builds up around your lungs and heart, causing coughing, shortness of breath, or an irregular heart beat. Fluid can also build up in the lower part of your belly, which can cause bloating.

You and your doctor or nurse can help manage fluid retention by:

- Weighing yourself at the same time each day, using the same scale. Let your doctor or nurse know if you gain weight quickly.

- Avoiding table salt or salty foods.

- Limiting the liquids you drink.

- If you retain a lot of fluid, your doctor may prescribe medicine to get rid of the extra fluid.

Eye changes

- **Trouble wearing contact lenses.** Some types of chemotherapy can bother your eyes and make wearing contact lenses painful. Ask your doctor or nurse if you can wear contact lenses while getting chemotherapy.

- **Blurry vision.** Some types of chemotherapy can clog your tear ducts, which can cause blurry vision.

- **Watery eyes.** Sometimes, chemotherapy can seep out in your tears, which can cause your eyes to water more than usual.

If your vision gets blurry or your eyes water more than usual, tell your doctor or nurse.

Clear Liquids

This list may help if you have:

■ Diarrhea (see pages 24 and 25)

■ Urinary, kidney, or bladder changes (see page 50)

Type	Examples
Soups	Bouillon Clear, fat-free broth Consommé
Drinks	Clear apple juice Clear carbonated beverages Fruit-flavored drinks Fruit juice, such as cranberry or grape Fruit punch Sports drinks Water Weak tea with no caffeine
Sweets	Fruit ices made without fruit pieces or milk Gelatin Honey Jelly Popsicles

Liquid Foods

This list may help if you:

- Do not feel like eating solid foods (see Appetite Changes on pages 18 and 19)
- Have urinary, kidney, or bladder changes (see page 50)

Type	Examples
Soups	Bouillon Broth Cheese soup Soup that has been strained or put through a blender Soup with pureed potatoes Tomato soup
Drinks	Carbonated beverages Milkshakes Coffee Smoothies Eggnog (pasteurized Sports drinks and alcohol free) Tea Fruit drinks Tomato juice Fruit juices Vegetable juice Fruit punch Water Milk (all types)
Fats	Butter Cream Margarine Oil Sour cream
Sweets	Custard (soft or baked) Frozen yogurt Fruit purees that are watered down Gelatin Honey Ice cream with no chunks (such as nuts or cookie pieces) Ice milk Jelly Pudding Syrup Yogurt (plain or vanilla)
Replacements and supplements	Instant breakfast drinks Liquid meal replacements

Foods and Drinks That Are High in Calories or Protein

This list may help if you do not feel like eating. See Appetite Changes on pages 18 and 19.

Type	Examples	
Soups	Cream soups Soups with lentils, dried peas, or beans (such as pinto, black, red, or kidney)	
Drinks	Instant breakfast drinks Milkshakes Smoothies Whole milk	
Main meals and other foods	Beef Butter, margarine, or oil added to your food Cheese Chicken Cooked dried peas and beans (such as pinto, black, red, or kidney) Cottage cheese	Cream cheese Croissants Deviled ham Eggs Fish Nuts, seeds, and wheat germ Peanut butter Sour cream
Sweets	Custards (soft or baked) Frozen yogurt Ice cream Muffins Pudding Yogurt (plain or vanilla)	
Replacements and supplements	Liquid meal replacements Powdered milk added to foods such as pudding, milkshakes, and scrambled eggs	

High-Fiber Foods

This list may help if you have constipation. See pages 22 and 23.

Type	Examples
Main meals and other foods	Bran muffins Bran or whole-grain cereals Brown or wild rice Cooked dried peas and beans (such as pinto, black, red, or kidney) Whole-wheat bread Whole-wheat pastas
Fruits and vegetables	Dried fruit, such as apricots, dates, prunes, and raisins Fresh fruit, such as apples, blueberries, and grapes Raw or cooked vegetables, such as broccoli, corn, green beans, peas, and spinach
Snacks	Granola Nuts Popcorn Seeds, such as sunflower Trail mix

Low-Fiber Foods

This list may help if you have diarrhea. See pages 24 and 25.

Type	Examples
Main meals and other foods	Chicken or turkey (skinless) Cooked refined cereals Cottage cheese Eggs Fish Noodles Potatoes (baked or mashed without the skin) White bread White rice
Fruits and vegetables	Asparagus Bananas Canned fruit, such as peaches, pears, and applesauce Clear fruit juice Vegetable juice
Snacks	Angel food cake Gelatin Saltine crackers Sherbet or sorbet Yogurt (plain or vanilla)

Foods That Are Easy on a Sore Mouth

This list may help if your mouth or throat are sore. See pages 35 through 37.

Type	Examples
Main meals and other foods	Baby food Cooked refined cereals Cottage cheese Eggs (soft boiled or scrambled) Macaroni and cheese Mashed potatoes Pureed cooked foods Soups
Sweets	Custards Fruit (pureed or baby food) Gelatin Ice cream Milkshakes Puddings Smoothies Soft fruits (bananas and applesauce) Yogurt (plain or vanilla)

Foods and Drinks That Are Easy on the Stomach

This list may help if you have nausea and vomiting. See pages 38 and 39.

Type	Examples
Soups	Clear broth, such as chicken, vegetable, or beef
Drinks	Clear carbonated beverages that have lost their fizz Cranberry or grape juice Fruit-flavored drinks Fruit punch Sports drinks Tea Water
Main meals and other foods	Chicken (broiled or baked without its skin) Cream of rice Instant oatmeal Noodles Potatoes (boiled without skins) Pretzels Saltine crackers White rice White toast
Sweets	Angel food cake Canned fruit, such as applesauce, peaches, and pears Gelatin Popsicles Sherbet or sorbet Yogurt (plain or vanilla)

Ways To Learn More

For more resources, see National Organizations That Offer Cancer-Related Services at www.cancer.gov. In the search box, type in the words "national organizations." Or call 1-800-4-CANCER (1-800-422-6237) for more help.

National Cancer Institute (NCI)

Find out more from these free NCI services.

Call:	1-800-4-CANCER (1-800-422-6237)
Visit:	www.cancer.gov
Chat:	www.cancer.gov/livehelp
E-mail:	cancergovstaff@mail.nih.gov

American Cancer Society

Offers a variety of services to patients and their families. It also supports research, provides printed materials, and conducts educational programs.

Call:	1-800-ACS-2345 (1-800-227-2345)
Visit:	www.cancer.org

Cancer Support Community

Dedicated to providing support, education, and hope to people affected by cancer.

Call:	1-888-793-9355 or 202-659-9709
Visit:	www.cancersupportcommunity.org
E-mail:	help@cancersupportcommunity.org

CancerCare, Inc.

Offers free support, information, financial assistance, and practical help to people with cancer and their loved ones.

Call:	1-800-813-HOPE (1-800-813-4673)
Visit:	www.cancercare.org
E-mail:	info@cancercare.org

fertileHOPE

A LIVESTRONG initiative dedicated to providing reproductive information, support, and hope to cancer patients and survivors whose medical treatments present the risk of infertility.

Call:	1-866-965-7205
Visit:	www.fertilehope.org

National Oral Health Information Clearinghouse

A service of the National Institute of Dental and Craniofacial Research that provides oral health information for special care patients.

Call:	1-866-232-4528
Visit:	www.nidcr.nih.gov
E-mail:	nidcrinfo@mail.nih.gov

Acupuncture (AK-yoo-PUNK-cher): The technique of inserting thin needles through the skin at specific points on the body to control nausea, vomiting, and other symptoms.

Adjuvant (AD-joo-vant) **chemotherapy**: Chemotherapy used to kill cancer cells after surgery or radiation therapy.

Alopecia (al-oh-PEE-shuh): The lack or loss of hair from areas of the body where hair is usually found. Alopecia can be a side effect of chemotherapy.

Anemia (a-NEE-mee-a): A problem in which the number of red blood cells is below normal.

Antiemetic (AN-tee-eh-MEH-tik): A drug that prevents or controls nausea and vomiting. Also called antinausea.

Antinausea: A drug that prevents or controls nausea and vomiting. Also called antiemetic.

Biological therapy (by-oh-LAH-jih-kul THAYR-uh-pee): Treatment to stimulate or restore the ability of the immune system to fight cancer, infections, and other diseases. Also used to lessen certain side effects that may be caused by some cancer treatments.

Blood cell count: The number of red blood cells, white blood cells, and platelets in a sample of blood. This is also called a complete blood count (CBC).

Bone marrow: The soft, sponge-like tissue in the center of most bones. It produces white blood cells, red blood cells, and platelets.

Cancer clinical trials: Type of research study that tests how well new medical approaches work in people. These studies test new methods of screening, prevention, diagnosis, or treatment of a disease. Also called a clinical study or research study.

Catheter (KATH-i-ter): A flexible tube through which fluids enter or leave the body.

Chemotherapy (kee-moh-THAYR-uh-pee): Treatment with drugs that kill cancer cells.

Constipation: When bowel movements become less frequent and stools are hard, dry, and difficult to pass.

Diarrhea: Frequent bowel movements that may be soft, loose, or watery.

Dry heaves: When your body tries to vomit even though your stomach is empty.

Fatigue: A problem of extreme tiredness and inability to function due lack of energy.

Healthy cells: Noncancerous cells that function the way they should.

Hormones: Chemicals made by glands in the body. Hormones circulate in the bloodstream and control the actions of certain cells or organs.

Impotence: Not being able to get or keep an erection.

Incontinence: Not able to control the flow of urine from the bladder.

Infertility: For women, it means that you may not be able to get pregnant. For men, it means that you may not be able to get a woman pregnant.

Injection: Using a syringe and needle to push fluids or drugs into the body; often called a "shot."

Intra-arterial (IN-truh-ar-TEER-ee-ul): Within an artery. Also called IA.

Intraperitoneal (IN-truh-PAYR-ih-toh-NEE-ul): Within the peritoneal cavity. Also called IP.

Intravenous (in-tra-VEE-nus): Within a blood vessel. Also called IV.

Long-term side effects: Problems from chemotherapy that do not go away.

Metastatic (MET-uh-STAT-ik): The spread of cancer from one part of the body to another.

Nausea: When you have an upset stomach or queasy feeling and feel like you are going to throw up.

Neo-adjuvant (NEE-o-AD-joo-vant) **chemotherapy**: When chemotherapy is used to shrink a tumor before surgery or radiation therapy.

Neutropenia: An abnormal decrease in the number of neutrophils, a type of white blood cell.

Neutrophil (NOO-tro-fil): A type of white blood cell.

Outpatient: A patient who visits a health care facility for diagnosis or treatment without spending the night.

Palliative (PAL-ee-yuh-tiv) **care**: Care given to improve the quality of life of patients with serious or life-threatening diseases.

Peritoneal (PAYR-ih-toh-NEE-ul) **cavity**: The space within the abdomen that contains the intestines, stomach, liver, ovaries, and other organs.

Platelet (PLATE-let): A type of blood cell that helps prevent bleeding by causing blood clots to form.

Port: An implanted device through which blood may be drawn and drugs may be given without repeated needle sticks.

Pump: A device that is used to deliver a precise amount of a drug at a specific rate.

Radiation therapy: The use of high-energy radiation to kill cancer cells and shrink tumors.

Recurrent: Cancer that returns after not being detected for a period of time.

Red blood cells: Cells that carry oxygen to all parts of the body. Also called RBC.

Side effect: A problem that occurs when treatment affects healthy tissues or organs.

Standard treatment: Treatment that experts agree is appropriate, accepted, and widely used.

Thrombocytopenia (THROM-boh-sy-toh-PEE-nee-uh): A decrease in the number of platelets in the blood that may result in easy bruising and excessive bleeding from wounds or bleeding in mucous membranes and other tissues.

Vomiting: When you throw up.

White blood cells: Cells that help the body fight infection and other diseases. Also called WBC.